D1860380

HÆMORRHOIDS AND HABITUAL CONSTIPATION

HÆMORRHOIDS AND HABITUAL CONSTIPATION

THEIR CONSTITUTIONAL CURE

WITH CHAPTERS ON FISSURE AND FISTULA.

By

JOHN H. CLARKE, M.D.,

SECOND EDITION-REVISED AND ENLARGED

GYAN

Published by

GYAN

Gyan Publishing House
5, Ansari Road
Daryaganj, New Delhi-110002
Phone: 011-47034999, 9811692060
E-mail: books@gyanbooks.com

Distribution Network
gyanbooks.com
India, USA, Canada, UK, Australia, France

© Publisher

All rights reserved. No part of this work may be reproduced, stored, adapted, or transmitted in any form or by any means, electronic, mechanical, photocopying, micro-filming, recording or otherwise, or translated in any language, without the prior written permission of the copyright owner and the publisher.

ISBN : 978-81-212-6695-6 (PB)
First Published, 1906

2nd Impression 2022

Printed at: Gyan Press, Delhi.

The book is sold subject to the condition that it shall not, by way of trade or otherwise, be lent, resold, hired out, or otherwise circulated without the prior publisher's written consent.

HÆMORRHOIDS AND HABITUAL CONSTIPATION
Author: JOHN H. CLARKE

HÆMORRHOIDS

AND

HABITUAL CONSTIPATION:

THEIR CONSTITUTIONAL CURE

WITH CHAPTERS ON FISSURE AND FISTULA.

BY JOHN H. CLARKE, M.D.,

CONSULTING PHYSICIAN TO THE LONDON HOMŒOPATHIC HOSPITAL.

Second Edition—Revised and Enlarged.

1906.

CONTENTS.

TO

THOSE EXCELLENT PATIENTS OF MINE

WHO, BY INSISTING ON BEING

CURED WITHOUT OPERATION,

COMPELLED ME TO BETTER UNDERSTAND MY ART

I Dedicate this Book.

PREFACE.

THE first edition of this work having been exhausted, I have taken the opportunity of putting it through a complete revision and adding materially to its contents. I have especially enlarged the portion relating to Fissure and Fistula, devoting a new chapter to each of these subjects—to every other part of the work I have also found it necessary to make additions.

The subject matter is of such vast importance that many volumes would be insufficient to exhaust its interest. In the absence of such, I hope my little work will do something towards stemming the tide of all-conquering surgery, and reclaiming for medicinal treatment its rightful and prior place.

JOHN H. CLARKE.

8 Bolton Street,
Piccadilly,
London, W.

January 30, 1906.

PREFACE TO THE FIRST EDITION.

ONE of the first things that proved to my mind beyond doubt the great superiority of homœopathy over the ordinary method of dealing with disease was its action in cases of old-standing constipation. In the early days of my investigation into the new system, I reasoned with myself, that if patients who had for years depended on purgative drugs for every action of the bowels they obtained could be delivered permanently from the necessity of using drugs of any kind, there was no longer any question which method I ought to choose. Such I found to be the daily experience of every careful homœopathist, and, following my preceptors I have proved the truth of it over and over again in my own practice. Some of the evidence I shall adduce in the following pages.

One particular object I have in view in writing this treatise is to demonstrate what homœopathy is capable of accomplishing in the world, if only it had fair play. That it does not have fair play many people know, but the majority do not. In every way possible the so-called orthodox allopathic school of medicine seeks to prevent the public and medical students from knowing anything about homœopathy, and puts all kinds of impediments in the way of medical men who would like to practise it. It may not be known that there exists a work much thought of by the allopathic sect, facetiously termed "A Code of Medical Ethics." One of the "laws" of this code begins with these words:— "It is derogatory to the true science of medicine to practise homœopathy." As well might it be said, "It is derogatory to true religion to practise the cardinal virtues." But we can see the force of the so-called "law" when we realize that the profession generally scorns the idea of *curing* patients, and only professes to *treat* them. Now, as Hahnemann pointed out, the business of a physician is not to *physic*, but to *cure*.

The best sphere in which to test the curative virtues of any system is in chronic cases. In acute cases there is more room for questioning the effects of medicines; but in old-standing cases,— tumours of slow growth and diseases getting slowly worse, or remaining stationary, or changing their phases but never disappearing,—here is a field in which the operation of a new factor in the shape of medicine is not to be questioned when a predicted change occurs, except by those who are wilfully blind.

The mere "physicking" of patients does not require the skill of a highly educated medical man; and I maintain that medical men should be above such work, except as a temporary expedient on occasion. There are times when it is worth while to obtain the physiological effect of some purgative medicine, but that is not a thing to put in the place of a cure. The constitutional cure of the condition is the only object worthy of the physician's aim. It is hardly possible to conceive the change that would take place in society if all medical men understood the power of homœopathic remedies. For one thing, our newspapers would be relieved of a large share of their advertisements. If medical men were educated to their true functions, quack nostrums would cease to have any vogue. Moreover, our landscapes and seascapes would lose disfigurements of which the artistic mind so bitterly complains.

Another object I have in view is to prove that the ordinary routine practice of allopathic doctors in trying to cure patients of piles by cutting them off is at once unphilosophic, injurious, and unnecessary. A large majority of cases of piles are perfectly curable by homœopathic remedies, and those which cannot be absolutely cured can almost invariably be so far remedied as to render operation out of the question. An operation does not remedy the state on which the piles depend; on the contrary, it merely removes an expression of the constitutional state, and if nature does not revenge herself for the outrage on some more vital part, the patient must be considered very fortunate.

JOHN H. CLARKE.

CHAPTER I.

HÆMORRHOIDS: THEIR NATURE.

SOME four-and-twenty years ago I received from a patient a very valuable lesson in the treatment of hæmorrhoids, which has been of the greatest service to me ever since. With the impatience of youth, the progress of the case seemed to me so slow, that I advised the patient, a lady past middle life, to undergo an operation. This she emphatically refused to do, and insisted that I should cure her by medicines; and I did. From that day to this I have not had occasion to advise operation in any case of the kind, in a large experience both in hospital and in private practice. I do not maintain that I have succeeded in curing all cases; but those which were not actually cured were so far benefited that no operation has been required.

And here I may say a word about the time required for medicinal cures in chronic cases. It was my impatience in the case I have alluded to that led to the suggestion of operative measures. The patient herself was quite willing to wait as the event showed. I am convinced that if medical men realised that hæmorrhoids are based on a constitutional state that is remediable, they would not so readily condemn patients to the surgeon's knife. But constitutional states require time for their change, and it is as ridiculous to expect to effect it in a short time, as it would be to expect a patient in typhoid fever to be well in a few days. And it must be remembered that though the ways of surgery are apparently more expeditious, *surgery never cures a constitutional state.* On the contrary, after a surgical operation the organism has to recover from the shock, and this may take a long time, and perhaps may never be complete. And this is especially true in cases like those of piles, where the constitutional morbid condition is left untouched by the operation, or is diverted to some vital organ. I have recorded such a case in my book on *Diseases of the Heart*, in which a fatal result followed such an operation. As the case is one of great importance it may be useful to give it here in full.

Sir S. E., a prominent Indian civilian, consulted me some years ago about a persistent cold in the head. Enquiring into its origin I found it had continued for about two years, dating from a time a little subsequent to an operation he had undergone for piles. The piles gave him but little inconvenience, but he was persuaded to have them "cured" by operation. Of course an operation never did, and never could, "cure" piles: it can only remove the hæmorrhoidal swellings without touching the constitutional condition on which they depend. The constitutional disease from which Sir S. E. suffered would be called "Psora" by Hahnemann, and "Gout" by other pathologists. The basis of gout (as I hope at some future time to show) is the psoric miasm of Hahnemann. Be that as it may, the operation was performed; the cold in the head came on—and something much worse than that. Noticing a peculiar quality in the patient's pulse, I made a cursory examination of his heart, and there found extensive degeneration of the aortic valves. On my putting one or two questions, but in such a way as not to excite any alarm, my patient said he knew his heart was all right, "*The doctors examined me carefully and said it was quite sound before I was put under the anæsthetic.*" Beyond giving general directions I said no more about it, as it could not have helped matters to have done so; but the sequence of events was quite clear to me. Before the operation he had no heart disease. The operation disturbed the morbid constitutional element, which at that time had a practically safe and innocent expression in the piles, and sent it in upon more vital parts of the organism. The chronic nasal catarrh and the diseased heart were the consequences. Sir S. E. only called upon me twice. A few months later I read in *The Times* that he had been found dead in his bed at a hotel in Edinburgh. I have no hesitation in saying that to operate for piles is as dangerous as it is unnecessary. Piles are not by any means difficult to cure by constitutional means, and when cured thus the *patient* is cured, and no dangerous after-effects are to be feared.

As another proof of the constitutional nature of piles, I may mention the case of a patient I once attended who suffered from very severe headaches. In her own experience she had found that a strong infusion of cayenne pepper would always relieve her headache, but with the invariable result of inducing an attack of piles. Here it is evident that the headache and the piles were merely different manifestations of one and the same constitutional state, which an operation could not possibly have relieved. To have "cured" this patient the operator would have had to remove the head as well as the piles.

Dr F. H. Lutze, of Brooklyn, records a similar case in the *Medical Advance* of May 1905: A married lady, 26, mother of two children, had tonsillitis with severe headache; the left tonsil more swollen and inflamed than the right; pain worse on swallowing saliva, but swallowing anything was difficult and painful. For this she had taken "Pepper tea," as she called it, meaning an infusion of Capsicum, which relieved the throat somewhat, *but produced severe burning and bleeding hæmorrhoids.* She received *Mercurius biniodatus* 200, which cured the headache and tonsillitis as well as the hæmorrhoids. Dr Lutze makes the same remark about this patient that I did of my case, namely, that for surgery to cure the patient the head as well as the hæmorrhoids would have had to be removed.

And yet the affection is completely given over to the surgeon in old school practice, as is shown by the most recent text-books on medicine. Pepper's *Text-book of the Theory and Practice of Medicine* makes no mention of hæmorrhoids as a disease for medicinal treatment. Quain's *Dictionary of Medicine* does, indeed, devote an article to the subject; but it is a surgeon who writes it, and though he gives advice for the internal and local treatment of mild cases, his general conclusion is as follows:—

> "External piles when large and troublesome, and internal piles when of such a size as to protrude at stool and to be subject to inflammation, ulceration, and frequent bleeding, *can be removed only by operation.*"

The experience of every careful homœopathist leads to a diametrically opposite conclusion, and one of the objects of this treatise is to demonstrate that piles are curable by constitutional remedies without any assistance from surgery.

That piles are not a mere local affair is proved, among other things, by the fact that they very often run in families. Gouty persons are especially liable to be troubled with them. In fact, piles are one of the commonest manifestations of gout. Moreover, piles are closely associated with the whole abdominal circulation, especially that of the liver. Essentially piles are a varicose condition of the veins distributed to the lowest portion of the rectum or lower bowel, with more or less hyperplastic growth of connective tissue. In this position there is a very rich network of veins which communicate freely with the portal and general venous systems. If piles occur outside the sphincter muscle which constricts the orifice they are called *external,* if within the muscle they are *internal.* Sometimes they are partly one and partly the other. Since, then, piles are essentially varicose veins (with a covering of skin or mucous membrane) they will naturally be dependent on the state of the venous system to which they belong. Now the veins of the internal abdominal organs belong to the portal system and discharge their contents into the liver. Any affection, therefore, of that organ which impedes the blood-flow through it, tells on the veins of the rectum, and may give rise to piles, or if piles already exist, may aggravate their condition.

One prolific source of piles must not be overlooked, and that is the habit of constantly taking purgative drugs for the relief of constipation. All varieties of pills containing aloes are very apt to bring on piles, and many drugs which are not purgatives (as in the Cayenne pepper cases cited above) will also do it.

CHAPTER II.

CASES OF HÆMORRHOIDS.

TO judge by my experience, there must be something in the atmosphere of the Houses of Parliament, or in the habits they engender, conducive to the production of hæmorrhoids as well as influenza, and the first case I will mention here is that of a prominent politician who consulted me some years ago.

CASE I.—BLEEDING HÆMORRHOIDS.

The patient was a tall, spare man, dark complexioned, between fifty and sixty years of age, who had travelled much about the world, undergone a good deal of exposure in open-air sports, and, without indulging to excess, was fond of a good dinner and his pipe. For five years, and especially for the last two, he had been much troubled with piles, which protruded, bled periodically, discharged continually a mucous fluid, and occasioned much heat, bearing-down sensation, and discomfort. The motions were at times constipated and light-coloured. The urine was thick after taking any wine. Without having actual pain in the liver he was often conscious of possessing that organ.

Before coming to me he had consulted his ordinary medical man, a well-known consultant in town, who had told him there was nothing for it, if he wished to be relieved of his trouble, but to make up his mind to lie up for three weeks and undergo an operation. As it was not convenient to lie up for three weeks just then—not to mention a possibly longer period—my patient, who had some acquaintance with homœopathy, determined to give it a trial. It was near the end of March when he called upon me, and I put him on *Nitric acid* 12. A month later he called again, and reported that he had been quite free from any inconvenience until a few days before his visit. He had been dining out, and had a little return in consequence, with constipation, but no bleeding and no bearing down.

℞ *Nux v.* 30.

After this I saw nothing of him till the following September, when he had a slight reminder of his trouble after a fishing expedition in which he had done a good deal of wading.

℞ *Calc. c.* 30, in powders, one night and morning. This kept him right till the following April, when *Lycopodium* was given, and he has had hardly any trouble since.

I will now give the case of the patient referred to in my introductory chapter.

Case II.—Obstinate Constipation; Marginal Pile.

This patient was a lady of very gouty family, past middle life. She had always been of a constipated habit, and had dosed herself freely with pills and other kinds of aperients. She had, however, partially escaped from the dominion of the latter by the aid of a domestic work on homœopathy, from which she learned the virtues of *Nux* and *Sulphur*, after which she had very little trouble in that way. I was called to see her for an attack of perityphlitis, and after she had got quite well of this, the attack of piles developed without any symptoms of constipation. There was a large protrusion, but in its origin it was partly external and partly internal, with great pain and discomfort. There was also some ulceration.

When I discovered the extent of the disease I came to the conclusion that it would take a long time to cure, and I then made the suggestion that an operation would be the most satisfactory way of ridding her of the trouble. But my patient, who was of a very sensitive temperament, was so terrified by the idea that I did not venture to repeat the advice, and though the complete cure did take some time, the acute symptoms were subdued in a few days by the internal and local use of *Hamamelis*, so that she was soon able to return to her ordinary avocations. *Æsculus* was given later with good effect. What remained of the pile was not so important as a return of the constipation, and it was whilst under treatment for this that the pile finally disappeared.

The origin of this patient's constipation is instructive, and may serve as a warning to those who have the care of young girls. When about fourteen years of age, she was sent to some friends on a visit. Whilst there, she was dreadfully constipated, and being very timid, said nothing about it. On this occasion she went eight days without an action. On another occasion when again on a visit, but to another place, the same thing happened; but this time she fainted, and when she revived she confessed what was the matter. Purgatives were there and then administered, and had to be continued ever after, till she came under the influence of homœopathy.

The medicine which I found give the most help was *Natrum mur.*, indicated by the largeness of the motions, and the feeling as if something remained in the bowel after the action. *Magnes. mur.*, *Hydrastis*, and *Lycopodium* also did good service, but it was not till *Natrum mur.* 200 was given that the condition was completely mastered.

I advised, in addition, the use of whole-meal bread, but that by itself had no effect, and, moreover, it had been tried before.

Case III.—Constipation and Bleeding Piles.

A governess, aged 30, consulted me at the Homœopathic Hospital on Nov. 9, 1887. She had been suffering from bleeding piles for nine months. She had never had them before, and attributed the attack to excessive walking and overwork. She was inclined to be constipated before the attack came on, and had been much so the last six weeks. Before coming to me she had attended at the Westminster Hospital. The bowel was then prolapsed, and had been returned by the doctor who attended her. He said, however, there was nothing to be done further but an operation. This so terrified her that she never returned, but came to the Homœopathic Hospital instead.

There was much aching pain of the bowel, worse at night, preventing sleep. The stools were large, hard, and knotty. Before the prolapse occurred she had taken a strong pill. The bowel remained in that condition for a fortnight.

℞ *Ac. nit.* 12, gtt. 1 quater die.

Nov. 22.—Very much better.

After this there was no more thought of operation. The medicine relieved her so completely that I saw nothing of her till the end of the following June, when I made this note:—

June 30, 1888.—Has been much better. Now only feels the piles when out of health. Motions regular. Feels weak, and is sleeping badly, waking at 4 A.M. Is constipated, which is very unusual; is very nervous. Frontal headache.

℞ *Ignat.* 12, gtt. 1 ter die.

July 4.—Very much better; feeling quite different. Feels worse in damp weather.

Repeat.

After this she saw me at rare intervals, and had *Nitric acid* 12 again and *Dulcamara* 12 (which always relieved her when feeling the effects of damp weather). She complained at times of pain in the left ovarian region. In February 1889, an abscess formed near the anus and broke, but healed rapidly under *Silica* 30. On April 10 of that year she had constipation, small green stools; this was relieved promptly by *Phosphorus*. All the time she continued to discharge her duties, which were heavy, and eventually she got quite well.

I will now relate two cases of an acute character.

CASE IV.—PILES FOLLOWING INFLUENZA.

A lady, who had recently recovered from an attack of influenza, suddenly, after stool, experienced great pain accompanying hæmorrhage and the appearance of a pile. The case being quite recent, and there being no complications, a short course of *Hamamelis*, given internally and applied as a lòtion, completely relieved and permanently cured the patient. The lòtion gave immediate relief.

CASE V.—ACUTE PILES.

This patient was so impressed with the relief obtained in her own case, that she came to consult me a short time after on behalf of a friend. This was a young unmarried lady who was subject to headaches, which had formerly been greatly relieved by *Lycopodium*. The attack of piles had come on suddenly *apropos* of nothing definite. There was, according to the account I received, a good deal of protrusion, with bleeding and pain. I did not see this patient, but I prescribed *Hamamelis*, and in a very short time she was well.

I may here say that *Hamamelis*, or Witch Hazel, has a very wide range of usefulness, in conditions of varicosis and piles. It has a very definite relationship to the venous system, and is one of the first medicines to be thought of where the veins are at fault. Of course it must be used with judgment, and cannot be expected to cure in all cases. Those cases which depend for their origin on some deep constitutional dyscrasia will require the appropriate remedies. *Hamamelis* may be given in almost any attenuation with good effect. For a lotion, twenty to thirty drops of the strong tincture to the pint. It may be used either cold or warm.

Case VI.—Rapid Relief of an Acute Condition.

As an example of what may sometimes be done in an emergency, I will mention the case of Lord ——, who came to me one morning in great distress, suffering from prolapsed piles, with excessive soreness and discharge, he having an important engagement to address a political meeting in the country the same evening.

Now there is one remedy which in my experience is more useful than any other where excessive soreness is the leading symptom, and that remedy is *Causticum.*

This I ordered him, with directions to take a dose every half-hour till relieved, and then less often until he returned. With this assistance he soon obtained relief, and was able to make a long journey and fulfil his engagement with very little inconvenience.

CASE VII.—PILES IN AN INFANT.

Prolapse of the bowel is not at all an uncommon occurrence in children, and is generally associated with constipation and straining. But it is by no means common to have a genuine attack of piles in an infant. This, however, did occur in an infant girl, aged thirteen months, whom I was asked to see. The little patient had been constipated since her birth, but the mother was greatly alarmed by the appearance of the swelling. When the case was described to me I expected to find prolapse, but on examination I found it was a genuine pile. *Sulphur* 30 was prescribed and in a very short time the pile disappeared.

Case VIII.—Bleeding Piles with Irritation.

An elderly gentleman, who consults me in the city sometimes, had an attack of bleeding piles some year or two ago. He is of a scrofulous habit, and as a child lost the sight of one eye from inflammation, and many years before I saw him he had fistula, which was operated on. When he first consulted me he was suffering from bleeding piles with a good deal of irritation about the parts, and constipation at the same time. His general as well as local symptoms pointed to *Sulphur*, and this gave him great relief. An attack of influenza interrupted the progress of the case, and when he was getting better of this a severe attack of bleeding came on and continued. Taking into consideration the constitutional habit of the patient, I prescribed a single dose of *Bacillinum* 100; the bleeding stopped at once, and though I have since prescribed for him for other ailments, he has never been further troubled with this.

When piles have continued for a number of years the tissues of the part—skin and mucous membrane—covering the varicosities become largely hypertrophied, and it is not always possible to reduce the hypertrophy by medicines. But it is almost always possible to combat the attendant sufferings, and reduce them to a minimum. If the power of the sphincter muscle of the orifice has been lost, it will be necessary to wear some kind of support, provided it cannot be restored. I will now mention a case of the kind.

Case IX.—A Chronic Case.

A gentleman, between 30 and 40, from the eastern counties, consulted me in the city a year or two back about his general health, and especially an indescribable lassitude impelling him to lie down frequently, even out of doors. In addition to this there was great sensitiveness to cold. Naturally active and athletic, he had never taken any care of himself. As a boy he had been troubled with ascarides. At school he used to over-eat, and would go for days without going to the closet. He also contracted other bad habits at school. His father had suffered from piles, and for five or six years the patient had suffered from them severely, with copious bleeding at times. His heart was not sound, being hypertrophied, and he was always conscious of having a heart. He had had a great variety of medical treatment. One doctor gave a strong preparation of nitric acid and purgatives. This treatment had the effect of causing severe hæmorrhage after every stool. The piles were large, and with every stool there was prolapse of the lower bowel. There was constipation. He contrived to have the action at night, so that the bowels might recover themselves when the horizontal position was maintained, but in the morning the protrusion had to be replaced and held in position by a support during the day.

Though now regulating his diet carefully, he suffered a good deal from symptoms of indigestion, especially flatulence. He had a tendency to bronchial cough. Most of the year he had wheezing at the chest, inclination to draw a deep breath, and a pretty constant expectoration of clear phlegm, which accumulated in the throat. He also suffered from weakness in the back.

℞ *Psor.* 30, four times a day. *Unguent. Hamam.*

This medicine had the effect of restoring his energy to a remarkable degree, the bowels acting fairly well whilst under its influence. In fact, the patient frequently remarked whilst under treatment that my medicines (which were all in infinitesimal preparations) had a marked tonic effect on him, without any of the penalties attaching to ordinary so-called tonics.

After this, *Causticum* 30, *Sulphur* 30, *Graphites* 30, *Lycop.* 30, *Alumen* 30, and some others were given with more or less benefit; but the prescription which gave most help was one of *Muriatic acid* 200 and *Graphites* 200 in succession, with occasional doses of *Bacillin.*

The result of the treatment was that though the piles had not been removed, the bowels were enabled to act satisfactorily without the help of purgatives, the piles were more manageable, and the general health very greatly improved.

Case X.—An Acute Case of Painful Piles.

A young lady, Miss C., wrote to me from the country on April 25, 1902, to send her something for piles, which she had had for ten days, but only for one day severely. They came on after riding horseback. I sent her *Hamamelis* 1, every 4 hours and a lotion of *Hamamelis* φ. Two days later I heard that she had had a good night but there was still a great deal of stitching pain through the anus to the left side, which was worse when sitting or lying, and better when standing. I sent discs of *Causticum* 30, to be taken every hour if the pain continued.

April 28, 1902.—"Ever so much better, but the pains came on so badly at lunch that I began the discs. Cannot sit up for long without pain." *Continue.*

April 30, 1903.—"Much better, but pain came on badly in the middle of the day. Bowels act regularly, but cause a good deal of pain. Period began on 28th, but has hardly come on at all. Cannot sit up for long."

℞ *Sulph.* 30 every four hours.

May 1, 1902.—(This report was written the day before the *Sulph.* arrived.) "Much the same as yesterday. Swelling gone down much in last two days. Pain comes on rather badly in middle of day, with intervals, from 11.30 A.M. to 2.30

P.M., but practically none before or after."

May 2, 1902.—"Very much better. Had very little pain. Sleep splendidly. Feel more like an ordinary person." Continue *Sulph.*

After this the patient was well.

CASE XI.—PAINFUL PILES.

Miss P., 30, consulted me in November 1903 for painful piles, which had troubled her since the previous April. The patient came of a gouty family, and had had a severe accident ten years before, which had caused prolapse of the uterus and swelling of the whole left limb, and when the swelling subsided it left a varicose condition of the veins of that limb which still persists. She had been vaccinated a second time two years before. She was a very active lady, but the condition of the left limb and the piles made it difficult for her to get exercise.

℞ *Thuja* 30, at bedtime; *Hamamelis* φ, for lotion.

December 27, 1903.—Piles have not troubled except on one day, when she did a lot of walking. Does not feel the leg at all. Veins better.

Repeat.

March 8, 1904.—Very much better in all respects.

From this time the patient was practically well till the autumn.

August 25, 1904.—For the last four or five days has been losing a slight quantity of blood with each motion. This has not occurred since last winter.

Repeat.

September 14, 1904.—Has been better. No more bleeding. Very much better; does not feel the piles at all now.

Repeat.

December 15, 1904.—Going on well. There is only a slight puckering discernable where the piles were.

℞ *Thuja* 30 and *Sulph.* 30 on alternate months.

July 6, 1905.—Practically well. Has been able to do a lot of walking in Switzerland. Veins not noticeable now.

Thuja has a very marked influence

on the rectum and anus; but in this case it acted as much by remedying the vaccinal element in the case as by its local action on the affected veins.

CASE XII.—RECURRENT PILES.

R. K., a barrister, 35, was cured by me of sciatica in the early part of 1904. In September of the same year he developed an attack of piles. He had some years before suffered from piles, which had been cured under homœopathy. He was very gouty, much influenced by damp. Had been three times vaccinated, the last time in October 1901; the vaccination had not taken.

September 27, 1904. Has been

troubled with piles for a fortnight. They are aggravated by walking. Good deal of stiffness in back and some pain down sciatic nerve.

℞ *Æsculus hip.* 3^x three times a day. *Thuja* 30 at bedtime. A lotion of *Hamamelis* 6 to be used after stool.

November 3, 1904.—Has been much better. Lately, there has been a return of pain in the back and down the left hip. Very hungry at 3 A.M.

Repeat.

December 6, 1904.—Has been much better. One day when there was snow he had pain. Piles bleed a little. 3 A.M., hunger gone.

℞ *Æscul.* three times a day. *Sulph.* 30 at bedtime.

January 19, 1904.—Has kept free from piles, and was well till the last three days, when there was a relapse, brought on by indulgence in wine.

I may say I had to reduce the allowance of alcohol for this patient to a minimum. He again received *Thuja*, and later *Lycopodium* 30 and *Urtica urens* φ. These kept him right, but indulgence in wine would always remind him of his troubles.

One great indication for *Æsculus* in these cases is "aggravation from walking." *Thuja* has also the same aggravation. It is also indicated when vaccinosis is an element in a case. The 3 A.M. aggravation is a further indication for this antisycotic remedy.

Case XIII.—A very Chronic Case of Piles.

Genl. R., æt. 56, consulted me first in June 1897. He had had piles for twenty years. They came first when he was stationed at Gibraltar. For the past three years they had given him much trouble, and in addition to the piles he had much mental depression. He had been treated with *Iron*, and one medical adviser suggested starvation diet, which did no good. There was a family history of suppurating cervical glands, and the patient had been vaccinated four or five times. There was a history of attacks of tonsillitis, and I found the pharynx congested. Appetite good. His drink is whisky-and-soda. Has smoked a good deal, but does not smoke now to excess. Is troubled with flatulence. Pulse irregular and intermittent. Heart sounds normal. Is chilly, and feels the cold much. Feet cold and damp. Sweats easily. Sleep good. He is better in summer, worse in cold weather; worse by walking, and worse after stool. I found a large purple pile protruding on the right side of the anus. This was sore when he sat down.

I ordered a course of *Sulphur* 30, followed by *Causticum* 30, and a lotion of *Hamamelis.*

July 27, 1897.—There is a good deal of protrusion. Piles come down on any extra exertion. Spirits fair. Sleep very good. Pulse 84, regular.

℞ *Nit. ac.* 12 ter die. *Bacillinum* 100, every ten days at bedtime.

After this date the patient removed from London and I did not see him again till May 1901. He had had a very trying time the previous winter. Walking and standing bring on the prolapse. I found the piles again very much in evidence.

℞ *Æsculus* 3ˣ thrice daily. *Æscul.* 30 at bedtime.

I explained to the patient that if he would let me follow up the treatment, I had no doubt I could do him permanent good, but not otherwise. To this he assented.

June 25, 1901.—Piles rather worse. Tongue white. Has not

slept so well. Good deal of depression.

℞ *Nitric acid* 30, 1 powder at bedtime.

Aug. 12, 1901.—Much less discomfort. Walking does not cause so much prolapse. Less moisture.

Repeat.

Oct. 17, 1901.—Has been going on very well. Very much less protrusion. On examination I found the piles much smaller. The patient had had a severe bereavement and was much affected thereby.

℞ *Ignat.* 30 every two hours, and later *Nit. ac.* 30 again.

January 17, 1902.—Bowels regular. Stools a trifle hard. There is prolapse after stool, but much less at other times.

℞ *Lapsana com.* ϕ. Three doses to go over two months.

March 20, 1902.—Steady progress.

Repeat.

June 3, 1902.—Going on well. Contracting power of sphincter better.

Repeat.

Oct. 22, 1902.—Patient came to see me. I found the patient's local condition very much improved.

℞ *Ranunculus fic.* ϕ, a dose every ten days.

January 5, 1903.—Has had ups and downs, but he does not think, on the whole, he has had so little inconvenience for a long time as during this winter, whereas winter is always his worst time.

Repeat.

March 26, 1903.—Very much better. Can walk better. On examination I found the anus looking normal.

Repeat.

June 20, 1903.—He again came to town to see me. His condition was so much improved that he was able to walk about London as much as he wished, without fear of bringing on prolapse.

Repeat.

Sept. 1, 1903.—About the same.

℞ *Æsculus hip.* 30, once a week.

November 28, 1903.—Going on fairly well till February 20, when he caught a bad cold which upset him generally, but did not cause any aggravation of the piles.

℞ *Lapsana* φ, once in ten days.

February 24, 1904.—I found the local condition very good.

Repeat.

September 30, 1904.—Going on well. I now interpolated three constitutional remedies, giving separately *Thuja* 30, *Sulphur* 30, and *Bacillinum* 30.

December 15, 1904.—Going on well, till a fortnight ago, when he had some worry.

℞ *Ranunculus fic.* φ.

March 1, 1905.—Much better for the last course.

Repeat.

May 16, 1905.—Very much more comfortable. The local appearance is normal.

Repeat.

I still hear from this patient occasionally. He is in an entirely different condition from what he was when he first came to me. Except for a little inconvenience immediately after the action of the bowels, he is quite well. This for a case of twenty years' standing is no small achievement. But it could not have been brought about without patient perseverance on the part of both patient and doctor. It should be remembered also that the general health of this patient improved, *pari passu*, with the improvement in the local condition. Indeed, in homœopathy, we can only cure local states by curing the *patient*.

CHAPTER III.

FISSURE.

FISSURE of the anus is often found associated with piles, though it quite as often occurs singly. It consists of a superficial ulceration of the mucous membrane in the form of a crack just within the sphincter muscle, and is accompanied by excessively acute pain. It is generally found in patients of a sycotic temperament, who are liable to similar ulcerations near other orifices. This, again, is considered by the old school as a purely surgical affair, and the treatment recommended is free incision through the centre of the ulcer. I shall show that this is an unnecessary proceeding: *fissure* is a constitutional affection, and is curable by constitutional treatment.

Case XIV.—Fissure.

Some years ago I treated a gentleman in the country who had long been a sufferer from rectal troubles, and had been treated variously for a variety of conditions, including salt-water injections for supposed worms. These injections had the effect of greatly aggravating his sufferings. On making an examination I found a fissure which accounted for all the trouble. The bowels were not at all constipated, —in fact the patient was very liable to diarrhœa, but the actions occasioned great pain nevertheless. His constitution was of the type described by Hahnemann as "sycotic," and by Grauvogl as "hydrogenoid," and as *Nitric acid* corresponded to this as well as the local symptoms, I prescribed that medicine, with the very greatest relief.

Case XV.—Piles Complicated with Fissure.

L. H., 42, Barrister and Journalist, consulted me on April 18, 1902, on account of piles, from which he had suffered more or less for eight years. Some months previously to my seeing him he had got run down through over-work, his digestion began to go wrong, and his piles became worse. They became complicated by *Pruritus* and attacks of violent pain, robbing him of his rest at night.

The patient came of a delicate family. His father, who is still living, is asthmatic. His mother was asthmatic, and died at 59 of phthisis. One sister had hip disease. He himself had always suffered from delicate mucous membranes. He suffered from violent and exhausting sneezing fits. He had had the uvula excised, a polypus and a piece of bone removed from the nose. He was liable to shivering, followed by sneezing fits, and readily took cold. His feet were inclined to be cold and slightly damp. His tongue was dirty. Appetite good for breakfast, but not good for other meals, though he had sudden sinking before lunch. Much flatulence passing both ways. Is liable to liver attacks. Whisky-and-soda aggravates his condition. The bowels are fairly regular, but he occasionally has to take Cascara. On examination I found a small fissure in the anus, a small pile protruding from the centre, and round the anus an area of skin looking like wash-leather, which I have often found present in cases of the kind.

Before coming to me this patient had been advised to go into a home, have an operation, lie up for three weeks, and he would be all right afterwards. It was not convenient to give up three weeks of his work, so he sought my advice. I told him that in my opinion medicines were quite capable of curing him, but surgery certainly was not.

℞ *Thuja* 30° at bedtime; a lotion of *Hamamelis* φ.

April 21.—After playing golf on the previous Saturday, had severe cutting pain in the rectum, which kept him awake at night. The next day he again played golf, and dined out the same evening. This night the pain came on before he went to bed. The pain was worse when standing or sitting. I directed him to go on with the powders, and ordered an ointment of *Graphites* 2^x ʒi to *Cetacean ointment* ℥i. This proved of great service to him in the subsequent treatment.

I now found it necessary to alter the patient's mode of living. During the greater part of the week he was working at full pressure, and his work was largely night-work. His duties frequently required him to attend public dinners, which invariably proved trying to his digestion. But neither of these were doing him so much harm as the exercise which he thought it was necessary for his liver that he should undergo.

Now exercise is a very good

thing for a man who has plenty of energy to spare, but it is a very pernicious thing for a brain worker who is spending all the energy he has to spare, and perhaps more, in brain-work. There are very few persons who are strong enough to do much of both at the same time. It is a different thing when a man is on holiday and freed from the strain of daily work. He can then put his energies into physical exertion without hurting himself—provided he does not overdo it. But it cannot be too clearly understood that exercise in itself is not by any means always a good thing. So I stopped Mr H——'s golf right away, and told him when he had an opportunity to rest both mind and body to take it. And as for his public dinners, I advised him to eat little and drink less. He soon found the advantage of following my advice.

May 1.—Has had a cold on him. Stools very hard and difficult; always perfectly firm; dark yellow, with slight loss of blood. Can stand and walk better.

℞ *Sulphur* 30, night and morning. In case of an attack of pain coming on, I ordered an ointment of 4 grains of Cocaine to one ounce of White Vaseline.

May 8.—Has been better. Cold has disappeared. Bowels act fairly, without pain. Cocaine ointment not required. Wakes heavy. Has stuffed feeling in the nose. Much sneezing.

Repeat Sulph.

℞ *Cepa* 30, discs, one every two hours, if required for colds.

May 22.—Very much better generally, but has had a chill from night work. Still wakes up heavy. Examination of the parts showed that the irritated appearance has much diminished. There was no longer any soreness in the fissure, and the pile was shrivelling.

June 2.—As a result of dinners and champagne obstinate constipation came on. Feels heavy and oppressed.

℞ *Nux v.* 3^x, every three hours, when required for constipation.

June 5.—Bowels acting more easily. Anus looks much better. Liver smaller.

℞ *Sulph.* 30, night and morning.

June 23.—Has had return of itching. Has had to take *Nux Vomica* at times. Bowels moved; stools small, dark, and greenish. Sleep fair. Appetite improved.

Repeat.

July 10.—Has been better. Bowels fair. Very little pain. Sleep good.

℞ *Psor.* 30, night and morning.

After this I did not see the patient again till November 7, 1902. He had been very well in the meantime, but a dinner had upset him, and brought on diarrhœa.

℞ *Sulph.* 30, and *Psoricum* 30, on alternate weeks.

March 10, 1903.—Has kept fairly well.

℞ *Sulphur*, night and morning.

April 28, 1903.—After two glasses of claret, had a severe attack of pain in the night. Abdomen distended, almost tympanitic.

℞ *Ran. fic.* 3^x, a dose every two hours. *Ran. fic.* ϕ, ten drops to half a pint of water, to make a lotion.

May 3, 1903.—Much better. I now gave the patient discs of *Nux v.* 3, with directions to take two of them immediately before and two immediately after a public dinner. This proved perfectly effective in neutralising the unpleasant effects he generally experienced after one of these functions.

May 27, 1903.—Has had much distention. A hot pain rises from epigastrium into the mouth. Recently not sleeping well. Has had a bad cold. Lost his appetite for tobacco.

℞ *Phosphorus* 12, night and morning.

June 8.—Very much better. He continued under this remedy till August 20, 1903, when I saw him for the last time. Since then he has continued well.

CASE XVI.—FISSURE.

Mr R. T., a professional man, about 50, consulted me on April 26, 1900, for excessive pain on passing motions. He was fair, tall, rather stout, subject to biliousness, with black spots floating before the eyes, but had good health generally. Family history good. He had been twice vaccinated, but it did not take much on either occasion. He was subject to colds in the head, which generally commenced in the throat. As a boy he used to have attacks of painful indigestion, and these were followed by rheumatism in the right arm. The bowels were his weakest part in youth. Once he had sunstroke. Has had malarial fever. Three or four years before I saw him he had piles. A year before he had much worry. At that time he had a slight pain in the anus after sitting on a hard leather chair. Six months later a stiff motion would cause pain. For the last three weeks has had much bearing down pain in rectum. Spirits depressed.

Tongue whitish; appetite very good. He is very fond of salt, but salt food makes him worse. Pulse 72. Sleep good. Feels better towards evening. Has some pain in the back like lumbago.

Has dry eczema between fingers and toes, which comes in Spring, and is worse when he eats salt food. Has warts on the chest which have been cauterised.

The bowels act daily about 9 A.M. He always had pain with the stool. An enema caused violent pain, and gave him eight hours of agony. I found the cause of the pain was a fissure at the right side of the anus. There were also some smallish piles. The necessary examination gave great pain, which he felt for some days after.

℞ *Nitric acid* 30, 28 powders, one night and morning.

May 10, 1900.—He was very bad all the first and second days; after that was better. Now has a good deal of bearing down. Feels as if the rectum was not fully emptied. Stools fairly easy. Dry feeling just inside sphincter. He is worse when standing and better when sitting. Pain in the back has gone. The cold in the head has passed away.

℞ *Causticum* 12, three times a day. *Hamamelis* ϕ for lotion.

May 16.—Pain has been worse.

May 17.—Soreness. Pain shooting up rectum, with dryness. Discontinue *Causticum.*

May 24.—Feels heart's pulsation in piles. Pain is now burning, there are no shoots. One day had agony to pass water. Stool greyish, tinged with blood.

℞ *Sulphur* 30, ter die.

℞ Suppos. cocain. $\frac{1}{4}$ to gr. v. cocoa butter. To be used when the pain is severe.

May 31.—On this occasion he gave me the following report.—Three days after the visit was the best day he had had for two months. The next day had a very difficult stool, with pain and burning. Next day a fairly easy stool; and the day after, diarrhœa. Soreness after stool. Eczema better. On whole a much better week. I found piles had developed externally on the right side of the anus in a figwart appearance.

Repeat.

June 9.—Is suffering from bile. Two days after visit had a very bad stool with blood, and after it the right leg felt numb. The stool is more painful, but the pain does not last as long after it.

℞ *Nux Vomica* 30, ter die.

After two courses of this the patient again took *Causticum* as prescribed on May 10, resuming the course interrupted on May 17.

On Sept. 4, 1900, I heard from him that this remedy, after causing "a copious flow of bile to assist digestion, seems to have done wonders."

I have seen this gentleman frequently since then, but not as a patient—he has remained well.

CHAPTER IV.

FISTULA.

IT is not an uncommon occurrence to meet with inflammation of the tissues at one or other side of the anal orifice. If this is not checked it may go on to the formation of pus which finds an outlet either into the bowel, or externally through the skin. In either case the tendency is to the formation of a *fistula*,—that is, an ulcerating tract leading from the original abscess to the surface, which continues to secrete a purulent fluid indefinitely.

Fistula has often been cured by homœopathic means, but it is much more easily dealt with if it can be taken in the abscess stage. The medicine that has the widest range in these cases is *Silica*. One curious observation I have made in regard to the action of *Silica* in these cases, which I do not remember to have seen mentioned by any one else. When an abscess forms at one side of the anus and *Silica* is given, very frequently the abscess will abort and *a new abscess will appear on the other side*, generally smaller than the first, and then both will rapidly get well.

CASE XVII.—FISTULA.

Mrs ——, 38, had consulted me occasionally for several years on account of constipation (for which she had previously taken Liquorice powder twice a week), piles, and other troubles, which had been entirely relieved by *Sepia* and other medicines. I had not seen her for four months, when she came to me on October 22, 1892. Ten days before, she had had a swelling on the right side of the anus, with very great pain at times, of a pricking, shooting character, and bleeding. The lump had gone on to the formation of an abscess and had discharged, and the discharge still continued. If the discharge ceased for a time, the patient felt ill and low-spirited. There was a pile on the right side, and on the same side a hard nodule, in the centre of which was the opening of a fistula.

℞ *Silica* 3, gr. ii. four times a day.

Nov. 14.—Has been much better. *Had a new swelling on the other side, but was better after it.* This appeared on November 8, and quite disappeared without discharging. Has had a good deal of discharge at times from the opening —sometimes mattery, sometimes blood. Has a sensation as if something were lodged in the bowel.

℞ *Sepia* 30.

This kept her right till the following March.

March 11, 1893.—Has had influenza and bronchitis, and the cough had caused the fistula to open up again. She was suffering from a scaly eruption on the face, acidity, indigestion, and pain about the abdomen from left to right after eating, and constipation.

Sarsaparilla was now given in a high potency.

March 25.—Bowels acting better; fistula much better; rash on face not so well; pains in hypogastrium and under left shoulder-blade.

She now received a course of medicines, *Alumen* 30, *Sulphur* 30, and *Psoricum* 30, given in succession in that order, with very great relief, in which the first named medicine seemed to have the principal share.

In June there was some return, and the same course proved effective. On October 11, she again had some difficulty in passing a motion, with bleeding, and a sensation that the passage was closing up. A local practitioner had strongly urged her to have an operation.

℞ *Sep.* 30, and *Nat. mur.* 30, on alternate weeks.

There has been no return of the old trouble, as I have ascertained from the patient, who called upon me years afterwards about something else.

With regard to the rash on the face, I may mention that the patient discovered she always had it after drinking Indian tea. China tea did not produce the same effect.

Fistula and Consumption.

The constitutional nature of fistula is so self-evident that it is not a little surprising that surgery should be resorted to in such a light-hearted way, as is generally the case. It is perfectly well known, even in the allopathic world, that a "successful" operation for fistula is frequently followed by some affection of the lungs. Fistula is frequently the expression of the consumptive state, and acts as a constitutional outlet. If this is treated by remedies directed to the constitution, the trouble can frequently be cured, and if it cannot, it is far better for the patient's future that it should be left uncured. It would be a somewhat different matter if surgery were regarded as the assistant of medicine, and if, both before and after the surgeon had done his part, the patient were submitted to a course of treatment directed to remedying the constitutional dyscrasia, of which the fistula is an outcome. But this is not the case. As soon as all *visible* disease-action is got rid of, the surgeon is satisfied, and as allopathic medicine knows nothing of constitutional cure, the patient is left with the idea that all has been done for him that art and science can compass. How far this is from being the fact the following cases, which show the relation between fistula and the consumptive state, will clearly illustrate.

CASE XVIII.—FISTULA AND PILES.

Mr E. C., 27, an engineer, consulted me on July 11, 1902, about a fistula which he had had for three years. He had been constipated all his life, and suffered from piles as well as fistula. He was tall and well developed, and except that his hands were cold and moist, he might be taken for a strong, healthy young man. But it is well for the physician not to trust too much to appearances. Enquiry elicited these facts of his family history. His father had died of Bright's Disease, and his father's father of phthisis. The patient's only brother had died of phthisis at the age of 16. His mother is living and in fair health, but her mother, still living, has epithelioma, and her father, who drank, died of an affection of the liver. It is evident that in this case the fistula was no mere local affair. The consumptive strain was particularly strong.

The patient had a good appetite, but he has an aversion to milk. The tongue was dirty at the back. There was a venous zigzag across the epigastrium, indicating portal congestion. The spleen and liver were both large. There was also some varicocele.

He had had measles and scarlatina in childhood, and a year before

I saw him had had jaundice. He had been vaccinated several times, the last time some six months before he came to me, and this time it "didn't take." The fistula made its first appearance in 1899.

The local condition I found as follows:—Internal piles which sometimes protrude. An indurated area on the left side of the anus which occasionally breaks and discharges. In addition to this there was the habitual constipation.

The vaccinal element, being the last taint introduced, was the first to be dealt with, and I prescribed a course of *Thuja* 30. Under this he was kept till Sept. 18. Bowels regular. Fistula getting larger. In the left crus of the penis is a thickening lengthwise, feeling almost like an encysted tumour. A little itching; no tenderness.

℞ *Silica* 30.

Nov. 3.—Slowly healing.

℞ *Tubercul. k.* 100, once in about ten days.

Dec. 10.—Fistula seems growing larger. More in evidence; discharges more readily, but not much at a time.

℞ *Silic.* 100.

Dec. 30.—Fistula better; he only feels it when piles protrude and are painful. Then the fistula is painful and discharges. There was a soft swelling towards left of anus.

℞ *Repeat Silic.* Ointment of *Ranulus fic.* ϕ, to be applied at bedtime.

Mar. 20, 1903.—Fistula less noticeable. Piles tend to protrude after stool.

℞ *Sulph.* 30, one powder at bed-time.

April 4.—Fistula scarcely visible. Piles rather prominent.

℞ *Ranulus fic.* φ, gtt. ii. in powder, once in ten days. Lotion of *Ran. fic.* φ.

June 30.—Has been pretty well till middle of month, when he had a chill and sore throat. I found the right tonsil rather big and the throat rather granular-looking. Fistula felt like a bit of gristle to left of anus.

℞ *Silic.* 100.

July 27.—Very costive. Piles and fistula very persistent. Fistula not so prominent, but longer and more sinuous.

℞ *Bac. test.* 30 at bedtime, three doses in the month. *Æsculus hip.* 30 the other nights.

This prescription was repeated on October and November. In January 1904 he had a cold and cough, and the piles were troublesome; but the fistula was much better, the thickening was disappearing. *Bacil. test.* 30, *Causticum* 30, *Sulph.* 30, and *Malandrinum* 30 were now given in succession.

Sept. 16, 1904.—Fistula a little troublesome.

℞ *Con.* 30.

Nov. 4, 1904.—Feels the fistula after cycling. Bowels rather costive.

℞ *Sulph.* 30.

Nov. 25, 1904.—Piles no trouble. Bowels regular.

℞ *Bac. test.* 100.

Jan. 27, 1905.—Fistula almost well. Piles come down at times.

℞ *Thuja* 30, three doses in the month; other nights *Æsculus hip.* 30.

March 31, 1905.—Fistula cured.

This patient remained at his work through the whole of the treatment. He was not incapacitated a day for the whole of the time; is constitutionally a different man from what he was at the beginning. In this case surgery would almost inevitably have directed the constitutional expression of his ailment to the lungs.

This patient had been for some time under the care of the late Dr Burnett before I took him in hand, and I may mention here the case of another of Dr Burnett's patients, whom I have seen, Captain C. This patient came to me for a patch of gouty eczema near the anus, and the history was somewhat interesting. Some years before, fistula had developed, and his local medical man (an allopath) sent him to a well-known surgeon, who advised operation without delay. Arrangements were about to be made when the Captain was advised to consult Dr Burnett, who said he could cure him without operation, and in no very great time he made good his word.

Some years after this, the said patch of eczema appeared, and Dr Burnett being no longer at hand, Captain C. again consulted his old adviser. "Ah," said he, jumping to a conclusion, "just what I said —the fistula has come back again. You will have to be operated on after all." And once more he was sent to the surgeon who had advised operation in the first instance. This time, the surgeon, who was not so hasty as the family doctor, was compelled to own that the fistula was absolutely and completely cured. "There is nothing for me to operate on," said he.

Case XIX.—Fistula in Patient of Consumptive History.

A young married lady, wife of a country clergyman, dark, *petite*, of consumptive type, first consulted me in October 1896, for troubles incident to pregnancy. This was her history:—For a long time she had suffered from post-nasal catarrh. Six years before I saw her she had piles and fissure, which were both operated on several times. Now post-nasal catarrh, piles, and fissure do not occur unless there is some constitutional dyscrasia behind them, and the business of the physician is to find out what that dyscrasia is, and remedy it if possible. On enquiring about the family, I ascertained that one uncle and one aunt had fistula. The uncle was operated on, and subsequently died of phthisis. The aunt refused to be operated on, and after several years the fistula healed, and she became quite well. When I saw the patient first, there was no rectal trouble, but she was constipated, her natural habit being one of relaxation. In April, 1897, the child, a healthy boy, was born. The following August an abscess formed near the anus, and this subsequently opened externally, a fistula resulting; or rather two fistulæ, one opening being near the anus and one near the coccyx. At this time she was under the care of the country doctor who attended her in her confinement, and he strongly advised operation. She was nursing her child all the time. The operation was declined, and Mrs C. again came under my care. *Silic.* 3 was prescribed in iii-gr. doses, and a *Calendula* lotion. The patient's general condition improved very much, and in April 1898 the coccygeal opening had closed, but the other remained open. *Bacill.* 100, *Maland.* 30, and *Fluor. ac.* were now given in succession.

The patient had a busy and somewhat arduous life, and the demands on her energies were greater than the supply, so that with her delicate constitution the strength was rather reduced.

Mar. 15, 1899.—Soon gets run

down in body and spirits. A little blood comes from one opening. Often much irritation just before the monthly period. Ulcers inside bottom lip close to the gums. These generally appear at the period. She used to have them constantly, but has been free from them for a long time previously to the last few months.

℞ *Teuc. Scorod.* φ, ten drops three times a day.

May 1.—Feeling better. Discomfort when the bowels act. Full feeling on the wound side afterwards.

℞ *Teuc. Mar. ver.* φ, ten drops ter die.

June 21.—Better. No inconvenience from the wound.

In November of this year there was rather an anxious period, as chest symptoms developed.

Dec. 20, 1899.—Hard cough, with pain on left side of chest on coughing. Three times little spots of blood appeared, and once thick blood in the expectoration.

℞ *Phos.* 3 every two hours.

Dec. 24.—Ever since the cold, has had full feeling in the left chest as if there was something to be coughed up. Often taste of blood in the mouth. Got up a little old-looking blood this morning.—I saw the patient on this occasion, and found the chest resonant. A little increased vocal resonance at right apex. No distinct dulness. A little pain in left apex. Cough was worse when lying on right side. *Continue.*

In a few days there was great improvement in all symptoms, and by the end of the month all fear of chest complications was at an end. A second pregnancy now followed, the child being born Dec. 1900.

The patient required a good deal of treatment subsequently to this, among the remedies given were *Therid.* 30, *Elaps* 12, *Bellis* 3^x, *Stephylococcin* 200. The result of it all is that the fistula gives no trouble, and the husband writes :—"Mrs C.'s health generally seems to have wonderfully improved, thanks to scientific medicine."

CASE XX.—RECTAL AND SCROTAL FISTULA AND ASTHMA.

This case, that of a city gentleman, Mr T., aged 48, illustrates in a no less marked degree the relation between *fistula in ano* and lung disease. In this case the fistula is associated with asthma, and when from any cause the discharge from the fistula is arrested the asthma is much worse.

Mr T.'s mother died of consumption when he was an infant. Twenty years before I saw him he had rheumatism, which began as writer's cramp in the right thumb. By the use of soda baths the pain was driven from the thumb to knees and ankles, and finally to right great toe. Eight years before he had stricture of the urethra, which was operated upon, and the result of the operation was that a fistula formed, discharging in the centre of the scrotum, beneath. In addition, there is a rectal fistula discharging near the anus. Appetite not good. Bowels act regularly. Liver and spleen both enlarged. The lungs were somewhat emphysematous. The asthma was always worse on Sundays, and was sometimes better in cold weather. Breathing was worse when lying down, and in the morning. His face had the dusky look of persons whose blood is not well oxygenated. The appetite was not good. Had pains round the abdomen after meals. He had been vaccinated in infancy only.

℞ *Tuberc. k.* 30, three doses to go over the month. *Urt. ur.* φ, gtt. v. in a wineglass of hot water every two hours when required for an asthmatic attack.

Oct. 30, 1902.—Very much better. Eats more than he used to do. After the first powder had asthma all day, but with the exception of a little "stuffiness" in the morning he was well till a few days back. Bowels act much better; stools black. Fistula discharges, but gives no trouble.

On these remedies he continued to make steady progress for some months. The asthma—which was his chief trouble, as it crippled him for the time being and rendered him unable to come to his business from his residence in the suburbs —kept in abeyance. In March, during the stormy period, his breathing was very bad. There was a good deal of wheezing in the chest, which was worse when he lay on the left side.

℞ *Thuja* 30, three doses in the month. *Urt. ur.* ϕ when required, as before.

Sept. 28, 1903.—Good progress was made up to this date, the asthma seldom troubling him, and the fistula being quite manageable. The report on this date was :—Not very well. For two days in the week asthma has been bad, making it impossible to lie down at night, the only comfortable position being standing, holding on to the bed-post. The drops (*Urtica*) cause him to sweat all over, especially about the genitals.. Fistula not discharging much. Bowels not confined.

℞ *Tub. k.* 30, once in ten days; *Lobel. acet.* ϕ, gtt. iii, in wineglass of water every two hours when required for asthma.

Nov. 10, 1903.—Twice had to take the drops, but the attacks were not so severe. He was able to lie down. The *Lobel.* did not relieve as promptly as the *Urtica*, but the effect was more lasting.

Repeat.

Dec. 17, 1903.—Scrotal fistula appears to be healing. Not so much itching as formerly.

Repeat.

Jan. 27, 1904.—Anal fistula appears to be healed.

Repeat.

April 15, 1904.—Had an attack of vomiting four days ago, and the next day severe pains under right breast, right arm, and below right scapula. Breathing caused pain, and he couldn't lie down any way. A local doctor who was called in said this was "severe congestion, but no pneumonia and no pleurisy." The discharge from the scrotal opening had ceased. The scrotum seemed filling with matter. The skin was inflamed and irritated, becoming sore when rubbed, and matter was exuded through it. He had found that when the first opening had closed, matter found its way along the urethra.

℞ *Nat. Sulph.* 30, every four hours. *Calendula* lotion to be applied.

April 19, 1904.—Better.

Repeat night and morning.

July 11, 1904.—No asthma. Right leg swelled last week. (I found it slightly œdematous.)

Things went on well after this under *Nat. Sul.* 30, *Bac. test.* 30, and *Thuja* 30.

May 10, 1905.—Patient wrote to me:—"The fistula seems to have closed up in part. Nothing comes through this way, but there is much swelling in the fork. Unable to walk."

℞ *Silic.* 30, every four hours. *Calendula* lotion.

May 17, 1905.—Very much better. Opening occurred in the night. Breathing much better.

Repeat night and morning.

Since this time the patient has had no real trouble. The anal fistula ceased discharging, and the scrotal one, which still acts as the constitutional outlet, is easily managed, and the patient's general health is vastly better than it used to be.

Case XXI.—Scrotal Fistulæ from Tuberculous Testicles.

Before leaving this subject I should like to relate briefly a case of fistulæ of a different kind.

Mr D., a Greek gentleman, 35, came to me on June 13, 1904, with fistulous openings on each side of the scrotum, communicating with swollen and tender testes. The history of the case was that he had recently been under an eminent surgeon, who had opened the abscesses and had recommended the removal of the testicles as they were, undoubtedly, tuberculous. This measure the patient objected to, and hence his visit to me.

He was a very delicate patient. His father had died of dropsy and his mother was melancholic. One sister had died of anæmia. As a child the patient had had depression, and there was a curious history of depression in the family. His mother had three sisters, and two of them suffered from melancholia. The patient had had influenza fifteen years before. Had malaria in Sidonia, the attacks coming on every eight days. Since a child he had had eczema at the back of the knees, on elbows, and on perinæum. The swelling of the left testicle had come on suddenly, as a sequel to influenza. The patient had never had any venereal disease, though he had suffered from nocturnal emissions. The surgeon who operated on him gave as one inducement to the patient to submit to castration that "in any case he would never pass semen again."

I told him homœopathy would give him a far better chance than surgery, and he put himself under my care.

℞ *Tuberc. test.* 100, three doses to go over a fortnight.

June 28.—Testicles very much better; less swollen; discharge ceased; no pain.

Repeat.

From this point improvement was steady and pronounced. On July 15 he reported:—"Fistula from left testis healed. Right fistula nearly healed." In August nocturnal emissions recurred, thus falsifying the surgeon's prognosis.

Sept. 9, 1904.—Has had cold in head. Throat was sore last week. Pain across eyes. Headache, with pain under eyes and in nose.

Bowels regular, slightly constipated.

Thuja 30, night and morning.

Sept. 30, 1904.—One week had headache over right eye. An abscess has burst without pain and is discharging.

℞ *Tuberc. k.* 30.

Oct. 24.—Swelling gone down. Right testicle nearly normal; left testicle has still much hardness in epididymis.

Repeat.

Nov. 21, 1904.—More discharge, but less thickening. Eruption better.

℞ *Bac. test.* 100.

Dec. 5, 1904.—Has had influenza again. Pain in chest some days. Testes tender.

℞ *Baptis.* 30, every two hours. *Repeat Bac. test.* 100.

Jan. 2, 1905.—Has been much better. Wounds closed. Eczema all gone. Left testicle still hard.

After this the fistula remained permanently healed, and the testicles steadily became more normal. He required no further treatment on their account.

CHAPTER V.

IRRITABLE ANUS.

A VERY common accompaniment of piles is irritation, affecting either the piles themselves or the skin in the neighbourhood. This may also occur independently of piles, and it may occur with or without eruption. More often than not it is of an eczematous nature.

CASE XXII.—IRRITABLE ECZEMA ABOUT THE ANUS.

A gentleman about forty came to me in the city, complaining

of a very troublesome irritation in the region of the anus, accompanied with discharge, with which he had been troubled for twelve months. On examination, I found the parts affected with an extensive eczematous eruption exuding a moisture. There was also a small pile with a cracked surface. A short course of *Graphites* with a *Graphites* ointment was sufficient to put this patient right.

Case XXIII.—Irritable Eczema.

Being called into the country to see a patient, I was asked, when there, to see the patient's maid, who was said to be suffering from boils, which were especially painful on sitting down. The young woman was in rather an unhealthy state generally. She was of a rheumatic habit, and was worse in cold or damp weather; subject to chilblains; and had multiple gatherings affecting the finger ends. Periods regular but scanty.

On investigating the so-called "boils," I found there were no boils at all present, but an angry-looking eczema with discharge. Four years before, she had had something similar. At the time I saw her both ears were affected with an eruption covered with crusts. *Mercurius vivus* 12, *Hepar* 30, and *Rhus ven.* 3^x, were successively given, and in a fortnight the ears were nearly well, and the patient was better in her general health, but the perineal discharge still continued, though without irritation.

Graphites 30 was now given with good effect, and since then this medicine has always kept her right in that particular when trouble has been threatened.

CHAPTER VI.

CONSTIPATION: ITS NATURE AND KINDS.

THERE is a widespread notion abroad, that if the bowels are not relieved once a day something dreadful will happen. This is one of the difficulties homœopathic doctors have to contend with when treating new converts for an acute illness. Circumstances alter cases, and under altered conditions it is not to be expected that all functions will continue to go on as before. Nor is it necessary. Therefore, the old notion that if the bowels do not act every day they must be punished and made to do so like disobedient children, is a relic of barbarism that must be done away with. Nature must be led and not driven if we are to expect curative results.

There is, however, a germ of truth in the popular idea. Given normal conditions, it *is* desirable that the bowels should be evacuated sufficiently at regular intervals. This is so far a justification for the pill-makers: it is only their method of remedying the difficulty, when such exists, that is at fault. Let us consider the conditions. The contents of a motion or *excreta*, as they are very properly called, consist of waste materials. They are not composed, as is popularly imagined, of portions of the food which are not digested. When food can be identified, it is an indication that the digestive process is imperfect, and constitutes a condition termed *lienteria*. Normally all the food is altered by the digestive juices, and taken up by the lymphatics and blood-vessels, which carry it to all the tissues of the body, and carry away from them the waste products which are incapable of any further useful combination in the body. These are passed off by the lungs, skin, kidneys, and bowels. But it is the mucous membrane of the intestines and its glands that separate the fecal matter from the blood-vessels, and it is this excretion which, with any absolutely indigestible substances that may have been eaten, constitutes the stool.

All the excretions of the body are poisonous, and if unduly retained are apt to set up poisonous symptoms. It is the same with the fecal matter: if it is not got rid of at the proper time, reabsorption takes place to some extent, with the result that many disagreeable sensations may be experienced, prominent among them being headache and malaise. In rare instances, as Dr Burford has pointed out, the use of an enema has brought on fecal poisoning in the shape of an attack of fever with eruption, lasting a day or two. The explanation of this is that the fluid of the enema has rendered the waste materials of the stool more soluble, and before the muscular coat of the intestine has reacted to the stimulus and expelled the motion, the mucous membrane has reabsorbed some of the poisonous material. Hence I say the popular idea that the daily action is a *sine qua non* of existence is not without some foundation of fact. But I hasten to add that it is not by any means universally true. There is no absolute rule in the matter. Constipation is an entirely relative term; every man is a law to himself. This may be laid down as a rule: However long a person may go between the actions, so long as the actions are without difficulty, and in the interval he experiences no unpleasant symptoms, there is no constipation. Many persons can go two, three, and even four days and longer, without any ill effect, and for them to worry their intestines with purgatives to obtain an action every day is the worst possible policy. Other people again, must have at least two motions a day to be comfortable; and so long as the motions are normal, they can no more be said to have diarrhœa than the others can to have constipation.

By the word "constipation" I understand the habitual retention of the feces beyond the time proper to the individual; or, difficulty or pain in the passage of motions, whether unduly retained or not.

Constipation may be due to a great variety of causes, and due regard must be had to these if it is to be successfully treated. Five leading factors in the physiology of the function are:—(1), The muscles of defecation, chiefly the diaphragm and the abdominal muscles; (2), the muscular wall of the intestines, and chiefly of the lower portion; (3), the mucous membrane of the bowels; (4), the secretions of the liver and pancreas which are poured into the bowel; and (5), the condition of the anal orifice. Defects in any one of these particulars may lead to constipation. All these elements are under the control of the systemic nerves, and nervous affections are often accompanied by constipation.

Heredity has often a great deal to do with the tendency to the disease, but there is no use in accepting morbid inheritances as if they were inevitable. If medical men were never able to remedy affections that are hereditary they would be of little use in the world. Irregular habits of life are responsible for many cases of the kind; improper food and drink, exposure and hardships for others, and for yet others, poisonous trades and improper medicines.

The varieties of constipation are endless, and attempts to classify them are not of much practical value. I shall illustrate a number of them in later chapters. Before closing this one, it may be useful to say a word on the terminology. "Constipation" and "costiveness" are generally used as synonymous terms. They may be used sometimes with slightly different shades of meaning by some writers but practically they mean the same thing. The word "obstipation" is used for cases where the degree is extreme. "Stoppage" or "intestinal obstruction" means some local mechanical interference with the passage of feces through the bowel. This is a comparatively rare condition, and is accompanied with a good deal of danger depending on the nature of the obstruction.

CHAPTER VII.

CASES OF CONSTIPATION.

THE cases already narrated have been for the most part illustrations of the power of homœopathy to cure constipation as well as piles, but I am going now to quote a few in which the constipation was the chief, if not the only, morbid condition.

CASE XXIV.—LIFE-LONG CONSTIPATION.

A married lady, aged about 40, who had suffered from constipation all her life, consulted me last spring about her general condition. She had taken all sorts of purgatives, including blue pills, and at the time she came to me was taking cascara in palatinoids. She had a feeling as if there was no power in the bowel. She had had an anxious life. Five years before I saw her a tumour was discovered in the right side of the abdomen and was still present. As there was cancer in the family this gave her some concern. She had a sinking sensation at the epigastrium in the forenoon, and some flatulence.

℞ *Sulph.* 30, three times a day; glycerine suppositories to be used in case of need.

In a fortnight the patient returned, and reported that she had had a natural motion every day without any additional help. From that time she had no occasion to have recourse to aperients. Shortly afterwards she went abroad, and on her return reported that she had managed very well. Sulphur was the chief medicine required for this trouble, though others were required for other conditions.

Case XXV.—Chronic Constipation.

This patient was also a lady, and was sent to me by a colleague in the country. She had been constipated many years, dating it from school irregularities. It is a point of great importance for the heads of schools to see that the scholars have every opportunity for forming proper habits. The neglect of this has entailed much distress among the pupils in after life.

Some years before I saw her she had had peritonitis when abroad, and this was followed by catarrh. By regulating the diet my predecessor had overcome a great deal of the difficulty, but not all, and when the patient came to me there was, in addition, a small pile and fissure. The patient was a great lover of salt. The tongue was coated. She had a bad taste in the morning; had a sinking sensation from 11 A.M. to 12; at times brought up mucus in strings. All her life she had been subject to hay fever.

Sulphur 30 was prescribed in this case also, and the only complaint she had to make was that *the medicine operated too powerfully*. The indication here was plain. The medicine was ordered to be taken at rarer intervals.

Case XXVI.—Constipation with Enlarged Abdominal Glands.

A young gentleman who had spent some years in Sydney was home for a time, and put himself in my hands in regard to his health on May 8, 1893. As a child he had been most delicate, and there was a good deal of delicacy in his family. His chief trouble was constipation, which he had had all his life, but worse latterly. The abdomen was not enlarged, but glands could be felt. Takes cascara in doses of from 20 to 40 drops. Stools in hard round balls, dark, nearly black. There was much flatulence, which he had great difficulty in passing.

I gave him *Opium* 30.

He returned in a fortnight, much better in general condition, but the constipation remained the same.

℞ *Bacill.* 100 *statim.*

Plumb. acet. 30 ter die.

To use enemata instead of taking purgatives. Glycerine suppositories.

June 24.—Better. Feeling very well in himself. Bowels acting more completely. Another dose of *B·cill.* Continue *Plumb. acet.*

June 28.—A good deal of flatulence. *Lyc.* 30.

July 1.—Better. Has felt better generally. *Rep.* In addition, one dose of *Bacill.* 100, and a few doses of *Carbo veg.* 200.

The patient continued to improve, and in about a week he had to sail for Australia. I prescribed a course of medicines for him, including *Nitric acid*, *Alumina*, *Lycopodium*, *Carbo veg.*, *Nux moschata*, and *Raphanus.* I heard later from his relatives that he became perfectly well.

Case XXVII.—Habitual Constipation.

About two years ago a gentleman, about 53, residing in the country, while on a visit to a relative of his, an old school consultant in Harley Street, took the opportunity of putting himself under my care. He was complaining of constipation, with tendency to bleeding and some irritation. He was at the time feeling somewhat out of health generally; had cold feet. Better out of doors and in cold weather.

I gave him *Sulphur* 30, and ordered him to use a lotion of *Hamamelis* after each motion.

In three weeks he reported himself as much better in every respect. His bowels had acted well. I repeated the prescription.

Here is a somewhat remarkable case published by me in the *Homœopathic World* of February 1885.

CASE XXVIII.—OBSTINATE CONSTIPATION CURED BY *Natrum Muriaticum* AND *Magnesia Muriatica.*

The patient was a young married woman aged 20. Nine weeks before the time of which I speak she was confined of her second child, and was then under allopathic treatment. She had made a tedious recovery, suffering from great general weakness, a vaginal discharge, headaches, and constipation. A fortnight after her confinement the doctor in attendance had given her an ounce of Epsom salts without any effect. She had suffered from constipation for so long a time that she hardly remembered when she had not. She usually had relief once or twice in the week by artificial means, but on one occasion she went for four weeks without a motion. The motions were very large, but composed of small lumps, and she had much pain after the motion. She had no piles. I gave her, on the 25th of October 1879, *Natrum muriaticum* 6, in drop doses three or four times a day. The following day the bowels were moved of themselves. She passed a large quantity of feces without pain, a thing she did not remember having occurred before. When the motion was passing she felt faint. Her health was much better in other respects.

On the 26th of November I saw her again. There had been no

return of the pain, but the bowels were again constipated. On the 4th of December she was in very good general health, but still constipated. The bowels were moved once or twice only in the week. The motions were large, long, hard, knotty, but caused no pain. I gave her now *Magnesia muriatica* 6, one drop twice a day. On the 1st of January 1880 I saw her again. The bowels were then being relieved quite naturally every morning. I saw her a long time after this, and learned that the cure had proved permanent.

I will now give the case of a lady from Johannesburg who was recently under my care.

Case XXIX.—Life-Long Constipation with General Debility and Sleeplessness.

Mrs —— arrived in England in thoroughly bad health. She always felt tired, and constantly wanted to lie down. She had been constipated all her life, and constantly had to take cascara. Never a good sleeper, she now suffered from persistent insomnia. Had cold feet, and was chilly generally. No appetite for breakfast, but wanted a meal at 11 o'clock.

When I saw this patient she was on the point of leaving for the Continent—so I ordered her a supply of medicine. *Sulphur* 30, to last her a good time. When she returned ten weeks later she was quite a changed woman. She was able to do without aperients; her appetite was good, and instead of having to be very careful, she had been able to eat like ordinary people. Her circulation was better, and her feet quite warm. The sleep was good, and her spirits also.

Nux vomica was the only medicine she required after this.

Case XXX.—Constipation with Excessive Menstrual Loss.

Mrs ——, also a Johannesburger, consulted me about her health in August 1897. She was the wife of one of the imprisoned Reformers, and had suffered much mental anxiety in consequence. For fourteen years, since the birth of her last child, she had suffered from constipation, for which she had taken purgatives and was now using enemata. When she took senna it caused prolapse of the bowel. She was also suffering from excessive losses at the monthly periods, which recurred much too soon. She had bad appetite, was nervous, and though of a happy disposition naturally, got very low at times. Complexion sallow and grey.

℞ *Nat. mur.* 30 four times a day. Under this medicine she steadily improved in all respects during the first month she was under treatment, and then it was changed for *Sulphur*. The first period was much more natural, and the second was altogether normal. She was a little thrown back by some worry towards the latter part of the time, when *Nat. mur.* again came in with good effect.

Case XXXI.—Constipation with Chlorosis and Dysmenorrhœa.

A patient of mine asked me to prescribe for her maid, aged 30, who had suffered many years from anæmia with its concomitant digestive troubles, and had been heavily dosed with iron in consequence. This had the effect of aggravating the constipation to which she had all her life been subject. She suffered excessively at each monthly period. Her pallor was extreme. The appetite was morbid, she craved indigestible things, and had much thirst. The spleen was enlarged.

After prescribing several medicines with but little effect, I gave, in view of the dysmenorrhœa and the probable sycotic origin of the trouble, a single dose of *Medor.* 200, and followed it with *Thuja* 30. A month later I had this report:—"Ever so much better. Getting quite a colour. Can *run* up stairs."

I will now give an instance of what may be done with homœopathy in cases that are in themselves hopeless. It frequently happens that cases of cancer are attended with constipation, and this may become the chief difficulty of a case.

I have seen cases of cancer of the rectum relieved again and again by homœopathy when purgatives or local treatment were quite out of the question. The case I will now relate was a case of cancer, but not of the rectum.

CASE XXXII.—EXTREME CONSTIPATION COMPLICATING CANCER OF VAGINA.

On Sept. 25, 1875, I was consulted by Miss ——, aged 50, who had been ill since the previous June, when she began to be troubled with a vaginal discharge. She took medical advice, and a cancerous condition of the passage was discovered. Three weeks before I saw her, some part of the growth had been removed by operation, and since then she had suffered so much pain that she had no rest night nor day. Bowels much confined; has had piles very badly since this illness came on. The periods had ceased for over a year. I found a very extensive cancerous growth in the vaginal wall, with a copious fetid discharge. The patient had a very bad family history, her father having died of cancer of the bladder. Whenever she sleeps she lies on her face. The last symptom, with others, pointed to *Nitric acid*, and I gave that medicine in the 12th attenuation every four hours, with doses of *Scirrhinum* at intervals. In a case which had developed so rapidly and to such an extent, it was not possible to hold out any hope of cure, but I thought much might be done to relieve.

The treatment was followed by great relief to the pain from the first dose of the *Nitric acid.* The offensive odour diminished very greatly. Slept well. At first the bowels were confined, and then they acted so much more easily that her friends thought the enema might be omitted. This was an error of judgment, for the trouble became worse afterwards.

About this time the patient having heard of the Cinnamon treatment of cancer, I was asked if I had any objection to her undergoing it. I replied that I had none, as I thought patients were justified in trying anything in desperate cases of the kind.

On Dec. 9, the friends came to me again and reported that though the cinnamon quieted the pain, its effect on the bowels was most unfortunate. They could hardly be got to act at all. The motions were like stones, and white as chalk. Piles very bad.

℞ *Alumen* 30 every four hours. *Scirrhin.* at bedtime.

Dec. 12.—Bowels wonderfully relieved on 9th and 11th; does not complain of any pain—only a soreness all over. Has slept well these two nights. *Continue.*

Dec. 16.—Not had any pain since 9th. Has slept well, and had proper relief. Only obliged to have enema once.

She died very peacefully on January 15, having been unconscious eleven hours. She had no more pain and no trouble with the bowels to the end.

CASE XXXIII.—INVETERATE CONSTIPATION.

Mr H. D., an unmarried gentleman, 47, consulted me on November 30, 1903, for constipation of thirteen years duration. He has to take every night one or two, and sometimes three, cascara tabloids. He had been farming in a southern colony for twelve years, prior to 1890, and latterly had lived in the Channel Islands. When at school he had gone a fortnight on one occasion without an action.

He had once had influenza; had been vaccinated three or four times, the last being in 1881. He felt well at sea. He was of fair complexion and bald. For twenty-four years he has had more or less nasal catarrh. He was subject to noises in the ears, and what troubled him most was an extraordinary sensation in the head at nights—just as he was losing consciousness—a sensation and sound as if clock-work went off in the head. This was very bad in the Colony, and began in 1884.

℞ *Sulph.* 30 on rising. *Nux vom.* 30 at bedtime.

I instructed him to leave off the cascara and use an enema if necessary, or a glycerine suppository, but not to trouble about getting an action every day.

Dec. 22, 1903.—Bowels act a little better. Had to use enema once or twice.

Repeat.

Jan. 15, 1904.—So far remedies seem to have some effect, but to-day was obliged to use a suppository.

℞ *Nat. mur.* 30 every evening at bedtime.

Feb. 11, 1904.—Since last writing had a motion every morning, though used a suppository on one occasion, as the stool was rather small and hard.

July 27, 1904.—Bowels act daily but not quite so well. Stools lumpy of late.

Sulph. 30, and *Nux* 30, were now ordered. This was followed by *Nat. mur.* 30, *Thuja* 30, *Ant. crud.* 30. All helped him, the last more especially, and this was repeated on July 26.

Sept. 8, 1904.—Have again been constipated, but had a stool practically every day.

Nat. mur. 6^x, gr. vi. 4, at bedtime.

Oct. 13, 1904.—Since last report has had no attack of the sensation in the head till a week ago. For twenty years has never gone so long without an attack.

℞ *Lycop.* 30 at bedtime.

Dec. 21, 1904.—"Every morning have had a perfectly satisfactory stool, not in the least constipated.

It is fifteen years since this happened consecutively."

Repeat.

Feb. 18, 1905.—His final report is as follows:—"It is now two months since I gave up taking any medicine, and I have had no return of the constipation, so I feel I am really cured."

CHAPTER VIII.

CONSTIPATION IN CHILDREN.

SOME of the worst cases of constipation with which we have to deal are met with in infants and children. Some children suffer a perfect martyrdom from it, and the ordinary method of administering purgative doses only aggravates the trouble. Much may be done by careful dieting in these cases, but they are only to be *cured* by specific constitutional medicines.

Children who have a tendency to enlarged mesenteric glands, "consumption of the bowels," as it is popularly termed, are very apt to suffer from obstinate constipation. I have frequently seen these cases completely relieved by *Plumbum*, especially the *Plumbum aceticum.*

Case XXXIV.—Constipation Cured by *Silica.*

A little patient, who gave me a good deal of concern at various times on account of her general delicacy, was much troubled with constipation, among other things. She got help from several medicines, but the one which relieved her of difficulty for long periods together was *Silica.* In this child's case there was prolapse of the bowel, and at times the motion would come part of the way and then *slip back again*, which is a leading indication of *Silica*. Its action was very prompt and satisfactory.

CASE XXXV.—VALUE OF MENTAL SYMPTOMS.

In order to show how necessary it is in homœopathic prescribing to look all round a case and take in the totality of the symptoms, I will relate that of an American young lady, aged 2½ years, who had come with her family from Venice, where they had made a prolonged stay, and who was then on her way home. She had always been constipated, though she once had diarrhœa, and after that the bowel came down. The stools were in hard balls and too large to pass. She passes blood with stool. Screams with pain, and wants her nurse to hold her. Is a bad sleeper; very restless; head perspires in sleep; grinds her teeth; has a croupy cough. *Nitric acid*, *Podoph.*, *Alumina*, were given with inappreciable result, upon which I took note of the child's mental symptoms, which I ought to have done at first. In addition to the screaming at stool, she would scream at other times, and not only scream, but scratch and bite if she got the chance. This pointed clearly to the peculiar brain irritation of *Stramonium*, and I ordered that medicine to be given.

This is the report I received—

the last before the family sailed. It showed clearly that the vital simillimum had been struck:—

"Better. Action sooner than expected. Though a hard stool, passed with much effort and crying, it was almost involuntary—not being able to leave the chair. No bad after-effect."

Case XXXVI.—Constipation in India-born Infant.

I will give just one more case, also that of a little girl of the same age as the last, just arrived with her mother from India. Her mother had been unable to nurse her, and she was constipated from the time she was put on cow's milk. Before leaving India she had an attack of diarrhœa, and for that was dosed with calomel. When on board ship the constipation again began. She was a fair child, and rather inclined to fatness. Head perspired at night. In India had a lot of boils. Her tongue was white; appetite variable. The motions were large, hard, healthy in colour. A little redness round the orifice. When she had the diarrhœa there was bleeding. She was fretful, though that was not natural with her. *Lycopodium* gave the patient very great relief. *Calcarea*, which was afterwards given, did much good, but did not relieve the constipation so well as the *Lyc.*

CHAPTER IX.

HINTS ON GENERAL MANAGEMENT.

THE patients who come to me have generally tried all known methods of diet, exercise, massage, etc., so that there is nothing much left for me to do beyond finding the right remedy. But I may make a few general remarks which may prove useful.

A moderate amount of exercise is a useful measure in slight cases of constipation, but excessive exercise is just as bad as too little. For city men who have to spend the greater part of their time in offices, to and from which they travel by train, it is a very good plan to select a house just far enough from their station to ensure a tolerable walk at least twice a day. There is nothing more dismal than your "constitutional" when it is a constitutional pure and simple. But by a little ingenuity it is possible to compel oneself to take a constitutional without knowing it. Horse exercise and cycling are useful, but cyclists should resist the temptation to overdo it. A good rule to bear in mind is: never to start on a ride *with* the wind, or *down* hill, if the hill is considerable. If that is done, the rider will probably go too far without knowing it, and the return journey will have to be fought *against* the wind or *up* hill, resulting most likely in over-fatigue. Whereas if a start is made against the difficulties, the rider contends with them when he is freshest, and has the easiest part of his work for the last part of his journey.

Allied to exercise is massage and systematic movements made under the guidance of an expert. These are both of great service where ordinary exercise from any cause is inadmissible. Abdominal massage is often effective in restoring the activity of the bowels, but unless it is assisted by medicines there is apt to be a relapse when it is left off. A rather peculiar form of abdominal massage is the "cannon ball" treatment—I cannot recommend it, though some claim great things for it. It consists of rolling a cannon ball (not too large, of course) round and over the abdomen whilst lying flat on the back before rising in the morning.

Hydropathy has a measure which I have seen used with success, I mean the towel pack. A towel wrung out of hot or cold (generally cold) water is laid across the body at night, covered with flannel, and fastened with another towel round the body.

Diet is a matter of great importance. Milk, eggs (especially the whites), jellies, gelatine, isinglass, are all constipating. Tea and coffee act in different ways on different subjects, producing constipation in some and looseness in others; cocoa is, so far as my experience goes, neutral, and may be safely used by all who can take it. Some of the thin varieties, as shell or nib cocoa, or Cocoa Essence, can be recommended; taken with little milk, though cream is admissible. White bread, whether it contains alum or not, is constipating to many people, and some of the excellent forms of whole-meal bread are much to be preferred, and should be used exclusively. There is no alum in them, as whiteness is not the object. Rice is also constipating, and arrowroot and milk puddings generally, and these should be avoided. On the other hand, meats and soups, fruit fresh and dried, vegetables cooked and raw, more especially green vegetables, oatmeal porridge and gruel, made with water, are relaxing. An apple or an orange before breakfast many people find of service.

Of late years it has become the fashion to drink quantities of hot water. Like other fashions this can be overdone. It should never be indulged in as a permanence, though it may be taken either night or morning for a time without much risk. The tendency is to relax and weaken the stomach.

It must not be forgotten that though the muscular coat of the bowels is composed of involuntary muscles, nevertheless the will has a good deal to say to the function. And if the call of nature is not felt at regular times, an effort should, nevertheless, be made at the time when the action should take place. Regular efforts made in this way will help considerably to restore lost or disordered function.

But after all is said and done about regimen and diet, there remain numbers of cases utterly uninfluenced by either, and if the daily pill or draught is to be dispensed with, some other medicinal action must be introduced.

On the local management of piles a few words may be said. When there is any trouble in returning prolapsing piles, or any suffering after the bowels act, it is well to encourage the bowels to act last thing at night. When there is any soreness, experience will tell that paper, even the softest, cannot be used. Water and a very soft towel are the only permissible cleansing measures. To the water, as I have said above, *Hamamelis* may usefully be added. Modern lavatories are so cleanly fitted up that there is no difficulty about a wash after an action. The pan can be emptied, and refilled with clean water, which may be used for bathing the parts. Hot water may be added if the cold gives pain; also the *Hamamelis*.

An ointment of *Hamamelis* applied at the time has a very soothing effect.

Sufferers from piles need not be told that all stuffed and heating chairs are inadmissible. There is nothing so satisfactory as cane-bottomed chairs for those who have any trouble with the rectum.

CHAPTER X.

MEDICINES.

BEFORE closing the volume, I may usefully add a few indications for the medicines most commonly called for in cases of hæmorrhoids and constipation.

Æsculus hip.—Blind piles, constipation, with lumpy stool, and pain in the back. Feeling as if the rectum were full of dry chips. I once permanently cured constipation in a confirmed morphia-drinker with this remedy. It is a very old custom among some country people to carry a horse-chestnut in the pocket as a preventive against piles.

Alumen.—Antidotes cases of lead-poisoning. Stools like clay-coloured stones. Bleeding with stool.

Alumina.—Paralysis of rectum. Stools hard and knotty. Even soft stools require great straining. Piles, itching and burning.

Bryonia.—Large, dry, whitish stools, evacuated with much pain. Headache worse on motion. Sensation as of a load in the stomach after meals.

Capsicum.—Protruding piles, with burning pain.

Causticum is a medicine which has paralytic symptoms prominent, and hence corresponds to cases where there is loss of power in the lower bowel. Soreness is a leading indication for its use in piles.

Graphites.—Useful in many cases of extreme constipation, hard lumpy stools; lumps often united with mucous threads. Piles; fissure; moist eczema, with irritation round anus.

Hamamelis.—I have said so much of this medicine in the text that there is little to add about it here. It is a safe medicine to begin with in any case of piles, and may be used internally and locally. It is especially valuable where there is much bleeding.

Hydrastis canadensis is a medicine which has proved very helpful in many cases. This medicine has cured many cases of cancer in its time, and it is a singular fact that many cancer patients are also constipated. A sluggish state of the bowels, inaction of the liver, light-coloured stools, piles, and indigestion with loaded tongue, are the indications for *Hydrastis*.

Lycopodium.—Hæmorrhoids or constipation; gouty, flatulent subjects. Urine deposits red sand. Symptoms worse in the afternoon.

Magnesia mur.—Conglomerate stool like sheep's dung. Pains in liver.

Nat. mur.—Chronic cases. Persons who have suffered from malaria and been dosed with quinine. Headache on waking in the morning, getting better later in the day. Inactivity of the lower bowel. After a motion it seems as if more remained behind.

Nitric acid.—Has a very wide range of usefulness in cases of constipation, hæmorrhoids, fissures, ulceration, and cancer of the rectum.

Burning, cutting pains before, during, and after stools are the chief indications for its use.

Nux vomica.—Especially suited to sedentary persons, inclined to be chilly. Restless, waking early in the morning, and falling into a heavy sleep later. A leading indication for *Nux vomica* is frequent urging, with inability to pass a motion.

Opium.—Obstinate constipation. Constipation with drowsiness. Stool in small black balls like marbles.

Phosphorus.—Constipation; stool long, hard, and dry, like a dog's. Piles. Pains darting up rectum.

Plumbum met. and *Plumbum acet.*—Aggravated cases of constipation; paralyses of the bowel, sometimes with very painful colic. A leading indication is an appearance as if the body were drawn in at the navel. On the other hand, many cases of "consumptive bowels" with large abdomen and inveterate constipation have been completely cured with this remedy.

Sulphur.—Piles and constipation in patients who are subject to skin irritation, acidity, headaches, intolerance of warmth, and sinking sensations, worse in forenoon.

INDEX.

L 2

Nanhi Shop
Online Shopping..
Www.nanhishop.com